Joachim Bonsack

Milestones in Modern Medical Research

Insights into a better Future

bup

Joachim Bonsack

Milestones in Modern Medical Research

Insights into a better Future

Print: ISBN 978-3-69035-200-0
eBook: ISBN: 978-3-69035-205-5

Order number: 1809 (Paperback)
Also available as an eBook

Bremen University Press, 2024.
The manuscript may not be used in whole or in part without the prior written consent of the publisher.

First edition December 2024

Bremen University Press
Fahrenheitstr. 11
D-28359 Bremen

bup@bremenuniversitypress.com
www.bremenuniversitypress.com

Joachim Bonsack

Milestones in Modern Medical Research

Insights into a better Future

Overview

1. GENOME RESEARCH	23
2. ARTIFICIAL INTELLIGENCE	47
3. IMMUNOTHERAPY	65
4. COMPARISON AND SYNTHESIS OF PROGRESS	77
6. SOCIAL IMPLICATIONS	82
7. OUTLOOK	85
8. CONCLUSION	89
10. INDEX	91

Table of contents

Introduction	9
Relevance of medical research	**11**
Dealing with infectious diseases	14
Combating communicable diseases	15
Prevention and management of pandemics	15
Technology transfer	16
Resilience of healthcare systems	16
Promotion of social stability	16
Innovation as a driver of progress	17
Strengthening international cooperation	17
New approaches to diagnosis and therapy	**17**
Increasing burden of disease	18
Limits of existing diagnostics	18
Challenges in therapy	19
Threat of resistance	19
Costs and access to treatment	20
Technological and scientific progress	20
Implications for clinical practice and society	20
1. GENOME RESEARCH	**23**
The basics of genomics and their significance	**23**
The Human Genome Project	**25**
Gene editing technologies	**27**
High-throughput sequencing (next-generation sequencing).	**30**
Clinical applications	**33**
Diagnostics and therapy of genetic diseases	**36**

Development of personalised medicine	40
Genetic modifications	43
2. ARTIFICIAL INTELLIGENCE	**47**
Introduction to AI in medicine	47
Relevance of AI in the healthcare sector	49
Current applications	50
AI in medical imaging	53
AI-supported therapy planning	55
Improved diagnostics and increased efficiency	57
Bias and interpretability of AI-models	59
Responsibility	62
3. IMMUNOTHERAPY	**65**
Scientific foundations	65
How immunotherapy works	67
Applications in oncology	68
Use for autoimmune diseases	72
Treatment of chronic infections	74
4. COMPARISON AND SYNTHESIS OF PROGRESS	**77**
Similarities	77
Differences	77
Assessment of relevance	78
Production, logistics and scalability	78
Ethical aspects	80
6. SOCIAL IMPLICATIONS	**82**
Social impact of new therapies	82

Accessibility and justice	82
Data protection and privacy	83
Responsibility and regulation	84
7. OUTLOOK	**85**
Synergies between genomics, AI and immunotherapy	85
Research gaps	86
Identification of further fields of application	86
Implications for medical practice	87
Long-term changes in the healthcare sector due to new technologies	88
8. CONCLUSION	**89**
10. INDEX	**91**

Introduction

In recent years, medicine has made considerable progress that has not only revolutionised the treatment options for individual diseases, but has also changed our entire understanding of health and illness. At first glance, these results seem to have little to do with each other, but there are in fact a number of red lines that show a beneficial and exciting connection that not only highlights the major achievements of recent years, but also points the way to what further progress can be expected in the near future.

This book is dedicated to presenting these groundbreaking developments that are fundamentally impacting our lives while paving the way for further innovation. It is a journey through the most exciting chapters of modern medical research, showing how closely science, technology and people's needs are intertwined.

From the decoding of the human genome to the use of artificial intelligence and immunotherapy - the advances covered in this book are not isolated from one another. Rather, they are interlinked, complement each other and reinforce each other's effectiveness. Genome research, for example not only enables a better understanding of the genetic causes of diseases, but also creates the basis for personalised therapies that can be developed more precisely and efficiently using artificial intelligence. can be developed more precisely and efficiently. At the same time, immunotherapy, which has already already enjoying considerable success in oncology, has the potential to be further improved through genetic and AI-supported research. These advances are exemplary of a new era of integrative medicine, in which disciplines work together across the board to solve complex health problems.

However, the significance of these developments goes far beyond technology. They influence people's lives on a deeply personal level. Diseases that once seemed incurable are now becoming manageable or even curable. Patients benefit from treatments that no longer rely on a "one size fits all" approach, but are customised to their genetic and medical characteristics. At the same time, these advances are changing the way we organise medical care and tackle health problems worldwide. From prevention to therapy, more and more tools are available that can be used not only more efficiently but also more fairly.

This book presents the most important achievements of modern medicine in a coherent, holistic context. It shows how these advances improve our quality of life and overcome existing barriers to healthcare. At the same time, it sheds light on how these achievements raise new questions and challenges - be it in the areas of ethicsaccessibility or sustainability.

By looking at advances not in isolation, but as an interconnected system, this book aims to help us understand the potential of modern medicine and open our eyes to future possibilities. It is aimed at readers who not only want to learn about the fascinating details of medical innovations, but also the big picture that drives these advances and makes them an engine for positive change in the world. Because one thing is clear: medicine is not standing still - it is constantly evolving, and with it the hope for a healthier and fairer future for us all.

Relevance of medical research

Medical research plays a central role in tackling global health problems that are exacerbated by demographic, social, environmental and economic factors. Given the growing world population, the increasing prevalence of chronic and non-communicable diseases and the threat of novel infectious diseases the importance of scientific advances in medicine is greater than ever. The relevance of medical research can be considered on several levels: preventiondiagnosticstherapy development, health policy and social stability.

Over the past 80 years, medicine has made extraordinary advances that have revolutionised our understanding of health and disease and significantly improved quality of life and life expectancy worldwide. These developments have been the result of a combination of scientific curiosity, technological progress and interdisciplinary collaboration, which has constantly opened up new possibilities for preventiondiagnostics and therapy.

The 1940s were characterised by one of the most significant breakthroughs in the history of medicine: the discovery and widespread use of antibiotics such as penicillin. This groundbreaking development saved millions of lives by effectively treating bacterial infections that were previously often fatal. Antibiotics quickly became a central tool of modern medicine, enabling more complex medical procedures such as surgery, transplants and chemotherapywhich would be inconceivable without infection control.

In the 1950s and 1960s, vaccination programmes revolutionised public health. With the introduction of vaccines against diseases such as polio, measles and smallpox, the global burden of disease was drastically reduced. In particular, the eradication of smallpox in the 1980s is considered one of the greatest successes of preventive medicine and proof of the effectiveness of globally coordinated health initiatives.

At the same time, technological innovations were driven forward in the 1960s and 1970s that fundamentally changed diagnostics and treatment. and treatment fundamentally changed. The development of imaging techniques such as computed tomography (CT) and magnetic resonance imaging (MRI) enabled doctors to look deep inside the human body without having to perform invasive procedures. At the same time, advances in pharmacology led to the development of effective drugs for the treatment of chronic diseases such as cardiovascular diseasehigh blood pressure and diabetes.

The 1980s and 1990s brought further milestones, particularly in molecular biology and genetic engineering. and genetic engineering. The discovery of the DNA-structure and the increasing decoding of genetic mechanisms laid the foundation for modern genome research. These developments culminated in the Human Genome Projectwhich was successfully completed in 2003 and enabled a complete mapping of the human genome for the first time. The resulting findings paved the way for personalised medicinewhich uses individual genetic profiles to develop customised therapies.

Over the last two decades, medicine has seen an even greater integration of technology and science. Advances in immunotherapy have revolutionised the treatment of cancer in particular by specifically training the immune system to recognise and fight tumour cells. In parallel, new technologies such as CRISPR-Cas9 have made genome editing have made genome editing more precise and accessible, potentially making genetic diseases curable in the future.

Another key area of modern progress is the use of artificial intelligence (AI). AI algorithms not only enable faster and more accurate diagnoses by analysing large amounts of data, but also the development of new medicines and the optimisation of clinical processes. In conjunction with the digitalisation of healthcare and the development of telemedicine, AI has the potential to make healthcare more accessible and efficient.

These developments mark the transition from traditional medicine, which focused on combating individual diseases, to integrative and precise medicine that puts people at the centre. The advances of recent decades have not only helped to improve the treatment of acute and chronic diseases, but have also laid the foundations for overcoming future challenges such as pandemics, increasing antibiotic resistance and demographic change.

In this modern era, where science and technology are seamlessly intertwined, medicine is faced with the task of combining the achievements of the past with the possibilities of the future. This transition to the present and future of medicine shows that we must not only build on past successes, but also actively work to make healthcare more equitable, sustainable and innovative worldwide. This book is dedicated to a detailed look at the recent groundbreaking advances that will shape the medicine of today and tomorrow.

Dealing with infectious diseases

Infectious diseases continue to pose a significant global challenge. New pathogens such as SARS-CoV-2 (COVID-19), but also well-known infections such as malariatuberculosis or HIVrequire continuous research efforts. Medical research enables the development of new vaccines, antiviral drugs and improved diagnostic procedures. For example, the rapid development of mRNA vaccines against COVID-19 was achieved through decades of basic research. These technologies not only offer short-term solutions, but also create the basis for future vaccines against other infections.

Combating communicable diseases

Non-communicable diseases such as diabetescardiovascular diseasescancer and neurodegenerative diseases are on the rise worldwide and place an enormous burden on healthcare systems, particularly in ageing societies. Medical research offers solutions by developing innovative treatment approaches, such as personalised medicinebased on genetic and molecular data. Advances in preventionsuch as improved screening programmes-programmes and risk prediction, are helping to reduce the burden of disease and improve quality of life.

Prevention and management of pandemics

Global mobility and climate change increase the risk of pandemics, as new pathogens spread more quickly and existing diseases are favoured by environmental changes. Research in the fields of epidemiology, virology and public health and public health is crucial in order to establish early warning systems and develop evidence-based measures to contain pandemics. Examples of this include international collaborations such as the Global Health Security Agenda network, which is supported by research to make healthcare systems around the world more resilient.

Technology transfer

A large proportion of the world's population has only limited access to modern medical care. Research is helping to develop cost-effective technologies that can also be used in resource-poor regions. One example is portable diagnostic devices that enable quick and precise diagnoses in remote areas. Research also creates the basis for global initiatives such as the "Access to Medicine" programme, which improves access to vital medicines.

Resilience of healthcare systems

The burden placed on healthcare systems by ageing societies, environmental disasters and economic instability requires sustainable and resilient approaches. Medical research provides models and strategies to increase the efficiency and sustainability of care systems. of healthcare systems. Telemedicine and digital healthcare solutions, which are driven by technological innovations, are playing an increasingly important role in ensuring comprehensive healthcare provision.

Promotion of social stability

Health is a central pillar of social stability. Epidemics and chronic waves of disease can exacerbate social tensions, deplete economic resources and promote political instability. Medical research helps to minimise such risks by not only treating diseases, but also providing long-term solutions to improve the health of communities. For example, the elimination of diseases such as polio has helped to promote socio-economic development in many regions.

Innovation as a driver of progress

Medical research is a driver of innovation that goes far beyond medicine. Technologies such as artificial intelligencegenomics and biotechnology have not only revolutionised medical practice, but have also influenced other fields such as agricultural sciences, environmental technologies and computer science. These synergies are helping to develop more comprehensive solutions to global challenges.

Strengthening international cooperation

Health problems know no borders and medical research is key to promoting international cooperation. Initiatives such as the World Health Organization (WHO) or cooperation on global vaccination programmes are based on scientific knowledge and research findings. These joint efforts strengthen the global healthcare system and promote the transfer of knowledge between countries.

New approaches to diagnosis and therapy

The development of new approaches to the diagnosis and treatment of serious diseases is of crucial importance, as existing medical methods often reach their limits. The urgency arises from the growing prevalence of diseases, the social and economic impact of health problems and the need to create personalised and effective treatment options.

Increasing burden of disease

The global burden of serious diseases such as cancercardiovascular diseasesneurodegenerative diseases and rare genetic disorders is steadily increasing. These diseases are not only leading causes of death, but also have a significant impact on the quality of life of those affected. The ageing population is also contributing to this development, as the risk of many chronic diseases increases with age. At the same time, newly emerging or mutating infectious diseases such as SARS-CoV-2 pose an acute threat that requires rapid and innovative solutions.

Limits of existing diagnostics

Despite enormous progress in diagnostics there are still considerable challenges. Many diseases are only recognised at an advanced stage, when treatment options are limited. Examples include cancers such as pancreatic cancer, which are often asymptomatic and therefore only diagnosed at a late stage. There is an urgent need for more sensitive and specific diagnostic procedures that enable early detection and thus increase the chances of successful treatment. At the same time, the increasing complexity of modern diseases requires the development of innovative technologies such as liquid biopsies, molecular imaging and AI-based diagnostic tools.

Challenges in therapy

The development of effective therapies is made more difficult by the heterogeneity of many diseases. Cancer-for example, is not a single disease, but a group of over 100 different diseases, each with different genetic and molecular characteristics. Standardised therapies are often not sufficient to cover this diversity, which makes the development of personalised approaches necessary. In addition, therapies for diseases such as Alzheimer'sParkinson's or antibiotic-resistant infections are reaching their limits, as the underlying mechanisms are not yet fully understood or there is a lack of effective treatment options.

Threat of resistance

The increasing resistance of pathogens to existing medications, especially antibioticsis one of the biggest global challenges. Multi-resistant bacteria can be deadly even in simple infections, and the development of new antibiotics is progressing only slowly. Similarly, resistance to antiviral and anticancer drugs significantly limits the effectiveness of existing therapies. New active substances and alternative therapeutic approaches, such as the use of phages or immunotherapies, are urgently needed to counteract this development.

Costs and access to treatment

Many of the therapies currently available, particularly for serious illnesses, are extremely expensive and inaccessible to large sections of the population. This affects not only low- and middle-income countries, but also developed countries where patients often suffer financial strain to gain access to life-saving treatments. Developing cost-effective and scalable treatment approaches is therefore a key challenge to ensure that medical advances benefit everyone.

Technological and scientific progress

While advances in genome researchAI and biotechnology offer promising opportunities, we are still in the early stages of utilising these technologies on a broad scale. The urgency to develop new approaches also lies in advancing these technologies to accelerate the transition from basic research to clinical practice. This requires not only scientific innovation, but also investment, regulatory adjustments and interdisciplinary collaboration.

Implications for clinical practice and society

Advances in medicine have far-reaching effects on clinical practice and society. They not only change the way diseases are diagnosed and treated, but also influence fundamental structures and processes in the healthcare system. In clinical practice, new technologies such as artificial intelligence and genomic approaches enable more precise diagnostics and personalised therapies. Thanks to genetic tests, doctors can better assess individual disease risks and develop customised treatment plans that are more effective and gentler on patients. Advances in immunotherapy and molecular imaging are opening up new ways of treating even complex or advanced diseases in a more targeted manner.

However, these innovations not only have an impact on medicine, but also on society. They help to improve quality of life by enabling diseases that were previously incurable or difficult to treat to be better controlled or cured. At the same time, however, they raise questions of equity and accessibility. accessibility. Advanced therapies are often expensive and are not equally available to all patients. This poses a challenge for the global healthcare system, as existing inequalities could be exacerbated if access to modern treatments is not expanded.

Ethical and social issues are also becoming increasingly important. Advances such as genome editing through CRISPR-Cas9 or the use of AI in medicine raise debates about how these technologies can be used responsibly. The storage and processing of sensitive medical data and the possibility of modifying genetic characteristics touch on fundamental questions of ethics and data protection. and data protection. These developments require close co-operation between science, politics and society in order to ensure that these technologies are used fairly and safely.

The economic implications are also considerable. While new drugs and therapies often entail high development costs, they could reduce healthcare costs in the long term by enabling more precise and efficient treatments. At the same time, new industries and jobs are being created in the field of biotechnology and medical technology. These advances therefore create not only medical, but also economic and technological impulses that shape society as a whole.

1. genome research

Genome research has fundamentally changed our understanding of health and disease. Since the successful decoding of the human genome in 2003, scientific breakthroughs such as high-throughput sequencing and gene editing technologies such as CRISPR-Cas9 have opened up new possibilities for researching and specifically influencing the genetic causes of diseases. These advances not only make it possible to precisely identify genetic risk factors, but also to develop personalised therapies that are tailored to the individual genetic profiles of patients. Genomics has the potential to transform medicine from a reactive to a preventative discipline and revolutionise the treatment of numerous diseases, from rare genetic disorders to cancer.to cancer.

The basics of genomics and their significance

Genomics is the study of the entire genetic information of an organism, which is stored in the genome. It involves analysing the DNA-sequences, their structure, function and interactions. At the centre of genomics is the goal of developing a profound understanding of the genetic basis of biological processes and deciphering their influence on health and disease. The decoding of the human genome in 2003 was a milestone that opened the door to a new era of medicine in which genetic information plays a key role.

The importance of genomics in medicine is demonstrated above all by its ability to understand diseases at a molecular level. Many diseases, especially genetic and multifactorial diseases such as cancerdiabetes and cardiovascular diseaseshave genetic causes or risk factors that can be identified through genomic analyses. This not only enables more precise diagnosticsbut also the development of tailored, so-called personalised therapies. Such treatments take into account the individual genetic characteristics of a patient and thus increase the likelihood of therapeutic success while minimising side effects.

In addition, genomics has has revolutionised preventive medicine. Genetic tests can be used to recognise risk factors for certain diseases at an early stage, even before symptoms appear. This enables preventive measures that can delay or prevent the development of diseases. Pharmacogenomicsa sub-field of genomics, also demonstrates its benefits: Here it is investigated how genetic variations influence an individual's response to medication. This leads to optimised treatment strategies that are individually tailored to the patient.

Another important field of application is oncologywhere genomics plays a central role in the identification of tumour markers and the development of targeted therapies. By analysing the genetic changes in tumour cells, specific drugs can be used to attack precisely these changes. This has revolutionised the treatment of cancer This has revolutionised the treatment of cancer and significantly improved survival rates for many types of tumour.

Genomics also has the potential to better diagnose and treat rare genetic diseases. Many of these diseases remained undetected in the past because their genetic causes were unknown. Today, genome research enables and the development of specific treatment approaches, such as gene therapiesthat directly target the underlying genetic mutation. underlying genetic mutation.

The Human Genome Project

The Human Genome Project (Human Genome Project (HGP) was one of the most important scientific endeavours of the 20th century and marked a milestone in biology and medicine. This international research project, which ran from 1990 to 2003, aimed to decode the complete sequence of the human genome and identify around 20,000 to 25,000 human genes. It was the first project to systematically map and analyse the human genetic code, providing a fundamental basis for modern genome research and personalised medicine. and personalised medicine personalised medicine.

A key success of the Human Genome Project was the creation of a complete reference sequence of the human genome. This reference still serves as the basis for genetic studies today and has revolutionised our understanding of diseases caused by genetic mutations. Before the project, little was known about the structure and organisation of the human genome. The Human Genome Project has shown that the human body is made up of a surprisingly small number of genes - far fewer than originally thought - and that the complex interactions between genes and environmental factors play a crucial role in the development of diseases. play a decisive role in the development of diseases.

Another breakthrough was the development of new technologies and methods that were advanced during the project. High-throughput sequencing technologies-bioinformatics tools and databases specifically developed for the analysis and storage of genetic information have revolutionised research. These innovations have not only advanced genomics but have also enabled applications in other biological and medical disciplines.

The human genome project has also had a profound impact on medicine. It laid the foundation for the development of personalised medicine, in which genetic information is used to make more precise diagnoses and adapt therapies to individual patients. In oncology in particular in particular, the project's findings created the basis for identifying specific genetic mutations that play a role in various types of cancer. This has enabled the development of targeted therapies that are now saving many lives.

In addition, the project has accelerated research into genetic diseases. It has identified thousands of genetic variants associated with specific diseases and opened up the possibility of developing genetic tests to predict and prevent these diseases. of these diseases. This was particularly important for rare genetic disorders that were often difficult to diagnose.

The human genome project was not only a scientific milestone, but also a social one. It has triggered worldwide discussions about the ethical, legal and social aspects of genome research. research. Topics such as data protection of genetic information, the possibility of discrimination on the basis of genetic characteristics and the limits of genetic intervention were intensively discussed and remain relevant to this day.

Gene editing technologies

CRISPR-Cas9 is one of the most important scientific discoveries of recent decades and has revolutionised gene editing. Originally derived from the immune system of bacteria, in which it serves to protect against viruses, this system was adapted by scientists for the targeted manipulation of the genetic material of cells. It allows precise interventions in the DNAby targeting, cutting and modifying specific sites in the genome. The technology consists of two main components: the Cas9 protein, which acts as "scissors" to cut the DNA, and a guide RNA (gRNA), which directs the Cas9 protein to a specific DNA sequence. After the cut, the cell activates its natural repair mechanisms, which can either lead to the inactivation of a gene or to targeted modification. This simple, cost-effective and highly precise method has enabled numerous applications in research, medicine and agriculture.

In medical research, CRISPR-Cas9 has created groundbreaking opportunities to treat genetic diseases. It allows scientists to directly correct mutations that cause diseases. Initial clinical trials are showing promising results in the treatment of diseases such as sickle cell anaemia and beta-thalassaemia, in which defective genes can be replaced by correctly functioning versions. CRISPR-Cas9 also offers the hope of a cure for hereditary diseases such as muscular dystrophy or certain forms of blindness by repairing the underlying genetic defects in a targeted manner. In cancer therapy the technology is used to genetically modify immune cells so that they can attack tumour cells more effectively. These developments mark the beginning of an era in which diseases can be treated at the molecular level by intervening directly in the genetic causes.

In addition, CRISPR-Cas9 has revolutionised basic research. It enables scientists to precisely deactivate or modify genes in order to study their function. This has deepened the understanding of fundamental biological processes and elucidated numerous disease mechanisms that were previously poorly understood. The technology is also being used to develop genetic models for diseases such as Alzheimer'sdiabetes or cancer which serve as the basis for the development of new therapies.

In agriculture, too, CRISPR-Cas9 has made enormous progress possible. Crop plants can be specifically modified so that they are more resistant to diseases, pests or environmental influences. In this way, higher-yielding and more robust varieties can be developed that contribute to securing the global food supply. The technology is also used to breed animals with improved characteristics, such as pigs that are resistant to certain viruses or cows that can thrive under extreme climatic conditions.

Despite the versatility and potential of CRISPR-Cas9 there are technical, ethical and regulatory challenges. One problem is so-called off-target effects, where the technology unintentionally cuts other parts of the genome. Such errors could have serious consequences, especially in clinical applications. The long-term effects of genetic interventions, particularly in germline cells that are passed on to subsequent generations, are still largely unexplored. This also raises ethical questions, such as the possibility of genetically modifying human embryos to create specific traits - a scenario often referred to as "designer babies". Such interventions could exacerbate social inequalities or enable abuse if the technology is not strictly regulated.

Another topic is access to CRISPR-Cas9-technologies. Although the method itself is relatively inexpensive, the development and application of genetic therapies are expensive, which harbours the risk that only wealthy societies or individuals will benefit from the advances. The international scientific community faces the challenge of developing standards and guidelines that both ensure the safety of applications and address ethical issues.

Despite these challenges, CRISPR-Cas9 remains a transformative technology with the potential to tackle some of humanity's most pressing problems. From curing genetic diseases to improving global food production and addressing fundamental biological questions, the possibilities seem almost limitless. Ongoing research will not only improve the precision and safety of the method, but also open up new fields of application. With responsible use and the development of appropriate ethical and regulatory frameworks, CRISPR-Cas9 could become one of the most influential technologies of the 21st century and fundamentally change the way we treat diseases and shape our environment.

High-throughput sequencing (next-generation sequencing).

High-throughput sequencingalso known as next-generation sequencing (NGS), has revolutionised the way in which genetic information is decoded and analysed. This technology makes it possible to analyse large quantities of DNA- or RNA sequences quickly, precisely and cost-effectively. Compared to traditional sequencing methods, such as Sanger sequencing, NGS is many times faster and more flexible, making it possible to analyse complete genomesexomes or transcriptomes within a few days. The introduction of NGS in the early 2000s marked a significant milestone that has revolutionised modern genome researchdiagnostics and personalised medicine personalised medicine.

NGS is based on parallel sequencing methods in which millions of DNA fragments are sequenced simultaneously.-fragments are sequenced simultaneously. The technology involves several steps: First, the DNA is cut into small fragments, which are then labelled with specific adapters and amplified. This is followed by sequencing, in which each DNA building block (adenineguanine, cytosine and thymine) is read one after the other, often using fluorescence-based methods. Sophisticated bioinformatics systems analyse and reconstruct the data in order to decode the entire sequence.

One of the greatest advances made by NGS is the drastic reduction in the cost and time required for genome sequencing. While the sequencing of a human genome as part of the Human Genome Project cost over a decade and around 3 billion US dollars, complete genomes can now be sequenced in a few days for less than 1,000 US dollars. can now be sequenced in just a few days for less than 1,000 US dollars. This development has made genome research accessible for a wide range of applications.

In medical diagnostics NGS has has enabled significant advances in medical diagnostics. It is now routinely used to analyse cancer genomes to identify mutations that specifically respond to certain therapies. It also plays a central role in the diagnosis of rare genetic diseases, where NGS enables the detection of mutations often overlooked by traditional methods. In addition, NGS has revolutionised the discovery and characterisation of microorganisms, facilitating the identification of new pathogens and the monitoring of outbreaks, as impressively demonstrated during the COVID-19-pandemic has impressively demonstrated.

The application of NGS in research has significantly expanded our understanding of biological processes. With RNA sequencing, scientists can analyse gene expression in cells or tissues, providing important insights into disease mechanisms. Epigenetic analyses, such as the investigation of DNA-methylation patterns, have also been made possible by NGS and help to understand the regulation of genes under different conditions. In oncology NGS has contributed to the discovery of biomarkers that improve early cancer detection and prognosis.

NGS is also a key tool in personalised medicine is also a key tool in personalised medicine. It enables the development of customised therapies based on a patient's genetic characteristics. For example, pharmacogenomics-tests performed with NGS can predict the efficacy and side effects of certain drugs, allowing for more precise and safer treatment. The technique also offers potential solutions for preventive medicine by identifying individual genetic risk factors for diseases.

In addition to medicine, NGS has also brought enormous progress in other areas such as agriculture, environmental sciences and forensics. In agricultural science, it is used to identify genetic markers for breeding higher-yielding and more resistant plants. In environmental sciences, NGS helps to analyse the biodiversity of microorganisms in different ecosystems. In forensics, the technology enables the analysis of minimal DNA-traces to solve cases more precisely.

Overall, NGS has fundamentally changed the landscape of genomics and the life sciences. It has not only deepened our understanding of genetic and molecular processes, but has also enabled practical applications in medicine and beyond. As the technology and bioinformatics continue to evolve, NGS is expected to play an increasingly important role in solving complex biological and medical problems. The combination of speed, precision and versatility makes NGS an indispensable tool in modern science and medicine.

Clinical applications

Genome research has revolutionised medicine and spawned a multitude of clinical applications in diagnosticstherapy and prevention significantly improve diagnostics, therapy and prevention. By understanding the genetic basis of disease and identifying specific genetic markers, doctors and scientists can develop personalised approaches that are more precise and effective than ever before. Genomic technologies, such as high-throughput sequencing and gene editing, have found their way into numerous medical fields.

One of the most important clinical applications of genome research is the **diagnosis of rare genetic diseases**. Many of these diseases, which were previously difficult or impossible to diagnose, can now be precisely identified by analysing the entire genome or exome. This enables not only an accurate diagnosis, but also targeted treatment and genetic counselling for the affected families. Exome sequencing has already helped to clarify the cause of diseases such as muscular dystrophy or certain forms of epilepsy.

In **cancer medicine** genome research has has brought about far-reaching changes. The analysis of tumour genomes makes it possible to identify genetic mutations that are specific to a tumour. This information is crucial for the development and use of targeted therapies that only attack the cancer cells while sparing healthy tissue. Examples of this are drugs such as HER2 inhibitors for breast cancer or EGFR inhibitors for lung cancer. In addition, genomics plays a key role in recognising biomarkers that enable predictions to be made about the course of the disease and the effectiveness of certain treatments.

Preventive medicine also benefits from genome research. Genetic tests can reveal individual disease risks even before symptoms appear. For example, women with BRCA1 or BRCA2 mutations may have an increased risk of breast and ovarian cancer. These findings enable preventive measures such as increased screening or prophylactic interventions. There are similar approaches for other diseases such as cardiovascular diseaseswhere genetic risk factors such as variants in the LDLR gene can be recognised at an early stage.

Another important field of application is **pharmacogenomics** which analyses how genetic differences influence an individual's response to medication. This information helps to select the right medication and dosage for each patient, thus minimising side effects and maximising efficacy. One example is the dosage of the blood thinner warfarin, which is influenced by genetic variations in the CYP2C9 and VKORC1 genes. Pharmacogenomic tests can be used to customise the dose in order to avoid complications.

Genome research has also enabled the development of innovative **gene therapies** made possible. These therapies aim to repair or replace defective genes that cause diseases. The first clinical successes are being seen in genetic diseases such as sickle cell anaemia and beta-thalassaemia, in which the underlying genetic defects are corrected. In ophthalmology, the gene therapy Luxturna has already proven that genetic visual disorders can be treated.

In infectiology genome research is used is used to identify pathogens more quickly and analyse their genetic properties. This is particularly relevant for the development of vaccines and antiviral therapies. During the COVID-19-pandemic, genome research played a key role in sequencing the SARS-CoV-2 genome and developing mRNA-based vaccines.

Transplantation medicine has also benefited from genome research has also benefited from genome research. Genetic tests enable a more precise determination of tissue compatibility between donors and recipients, which increases the success rate of organ transplants. Research is also being conducted into how genetic factors influence the immune response in order to better control rejection reactions.

Genome research has also enabled significant advances in **mental health**. Studies on the genetic architecture of disorders such as depression, schizophrenia and autism have helped to identify complex genetic risk factors. These findings could lead to new diagnostic tools and personalised treatments in the future.

In **pregnancy and prenatal diagnostics**, genome research has also brought has also brought ground-breaking progress. Non-invasive prenatal tests (NIPT), which are based on the analysis of cell-free foetal DNA in the mother's blood, enable the early detection of genetic anomalies such as trisomy 21 without having to perform invasive procedures such as amniocentesis without having to carry out invasive procedures such as amniocentesis.

Diagnostics and therapy of genetic diseases

The diagnosis and therapy of genetic diseases have undergone a profound transformation due to advances in genome research. have undergone a profound transformation. Genetic diseases caused by mutations in single or multiple genes often pose complex diagnostic and therapeutic challenges. Thanks to modern genomic technologies such as high-throughput sequencing (next-generation sequencing, NGS) and gene editing, these diseases can now be diagnosed more precisely and treated in a targeted manner.

In the **diagnosis** of genetic diseases, genome research has has initiated a paradigm shift. Traditional diagnostic methods, such as individual molecular genetic tests, were often time-consuming and could only recognise specific mutations. With NGS it is now possible to analyse the entire genome (WGS, Whole Genome sequencing) or exome (WES, Whole Exome sequencing) of a patient in a short time and at a reasonable cost. This makes it possible to comprehensively analyse the genetic causes of diseases, even in patients with unspecific or complex symptoms. Exome sequencing is often used to identify rare genetic diseases in which a large number of potential genes could be affected. One example is muscular dystrophy, where mutations in several different genes may be the cause. Genome analysis can also be used to discover new genetic variants that reveal previously unknown disease mechanisms.

The diagnosis of of genetic diseases is supplemented by precise genetic tests that target specific mutations. For example, carriers of genetic mutations such as BRCA1 or BRCA2, which increase the risk of breast and ovarian cancer, can be identified through targeted tests. Such diagnoses are important not only for the patient, but also for family members who may be at increased risk of the same mutations.

In the **treatment of** genetic diseases, genome research has also has also made ground-breaking progress possible. Gene therapies are one of the most promising developments in this field. They aim to directly correct or replace faulty genes. One example is gene therapy for severe hereditary retinal diseases such as Leber's congenital amaurosis, in which the defective RPE65 gene is replaced by a functional gene. Luxturnaan approved gene therapy, has shown that such approaches can restore patients' vision.

Another example is the treatment of sickle cell anaemia and beta-thalassaemia, which are caused by faulty haemoglobin genes. Through the use of gene editing technologies such as CRISPR-Cas9 the faulty genes can be precisely corrected, which has the potential to permanently cure these diseases. Initial clinical trials with CRISPR-based gene therapy are showing promising results and could represent a future standard in the treatment of genetic diseases.

In addition to gene therapy, genome research has has also driven the development of specific drugs that target genetic mechanisms. One example is the development of drugs for cystic fibrosisthat improve the function of the mutated CFTR gene. These drugs, such as ivacaftoraddress the molecular causes of the disease and have significantly improved the quality of life and life expectancy of patients.

The prenatal diagnosis of genetic diseases has also made significant progress has also made significant progress. Non-invasive prenatal tests (NIPT) analyse cell-free fetal DNA in the mother's blood and enable the early detection of genetic anomalies such as trisomy 21without the risk of invasive procedures. This has significantly increased the safety and accuracy of prenatal diagnoses and gives parents and doctors more room for manoeuvre.

Despite the impressive progress, there are still challenges. One of these is the interpretation of genetic data, particularly in the case of variants of unknown clinical significance. Not all genetic mutations necessarily lead to disease, and the clinical significance of many genetic variants remains unclear. This requires the integration of genomic data with other diagnostic information in order to make informed decisions. In addition, the ethical dimension of genetic diagnostics and and therapy poses a challenge. The handling of genetic information requires strict data protection guidelines, and the possibility of manipulating germline cells raises social and ethical questions.

The diagnosis and therapy of genetic diseases have entered a new era through genome research. has ushered in a new era. The ability to precisely identify and specifically treat genetic causes offers hope for patients who could previously only be treated symptomatically. With the ongoing development of genomic technologies and gene therapies there is great potential to better understand and effectively treat a wide range of genetic diseases, which will sustainably improve healthcare and quality of life for millions of people worldwide.

Development of personalised medicine

Personalised medicinealso known as precision medicine, has undergone a transformative development through advances in genome research and the utilisation of genetic profiles. The aim of personalised medicine is to tailor diagnoses, prevention strategies and therapies to the individual genetic, molecular and clinical characteristics of each patient. In contrast to conventional approaches, which provide standardised treatments for all patients, personalised medicine uses detailed genetic information to develop the best possible therapy for each individual. This increases the effectiveness of treatment, minimises side effects and opens up new possibilities in the prevention and cure of complex diseases. and cure complex diseases.

The basis of personalised medicine is the analysis of individual genetic profiles, which is made possible by technologies such as high-throughput sequencing (next-generation sequencing, NGS). (next-generation sequencing, NGS) and bioinformatic analyses. These methods make it possible to identify genetic variations that are responsible for the development of disease or the response to medication. For example, mutations in certain genes, such as BRCA1 and BRCA2, can significantly increase the risk of breast and ovarian cancer. With this knowledge, preventive measures such as close monitoring or prophylactic operations can be planned individually.

In cancer therapy personalised medicine has has made remarkable progress. Tumour DNA-analyses can identify specific genetic mutations that drive tumour growth. These findings enable the use of targeted therapies that act specifically against these mutations, such as EGFR inhibitors for lung cancer or HER2 inhibitors for breast cancer. Such therapies are often more effective and gentler than conventional chemotherapiesas they attack the tumour tissue precisely and largely spare healthy tissue. The analysis of tumour DNA has also enabled the development of so-called liquid biopsies, in which genetic information is obtained from circulating tumour DNA in the blood. This non-invasive method offers a quick and safe way of monitoring the progression of the disease and adapting the therapy.

Another key field of application for personalised medicine is pharmacogenomics. This investigates how genetic variations influence an individual's response to medication. Some patients metabolise drugs faster or slower due to genetic differences, which influences their effectiveness or the risk of side effects. For example, variants in the CYP2C19 gene affect the efficacy of clopidogrela blood thinner that is often prescribed after heart attacks. Genetic testing makes it possible to choose alternative drugs or dosages that are better suited to the individual needs of the patient. Such approaches not only improve the safety and effectiveness of treatment, but also help to reduce healthcare costs by avoiding ineffective therapies.

Personalised medicine has also made significant progress in the treatment of genetic diseases such as cystic fibrosis or sickle cell anaemiahave also made progress. The identification of specific genetic defects has led to the development of targeted therapies that act at the molecular level. One example is ivacaftora drug that improves the function of the mutated CFTR protein in cystic fibrosis patients with certain mutations. These therapeutic approaches illustrate how genetic profiles can be used to develop treatments for specific patient groups.

In addition, personalised medicine opens up opens up new possibilities in preventive medicine. Genetic tests can be used to minimise the risk of chronic diseases such as diabetescardiovascular diseases or neurodegenerative diseases such as Alzheimer's at an early stage. This knowledge makes it possible to customise preventive measures such as lifestyle changes or regular check-ups in order to reduce the risk of disease or delay its onset.

However, developments in personalised medicine also pose challenges. The interpretation of genetic data requires specialised expertise and bioinformatic analyses, which are associated with high costs. In addition, not all genetic variations are fully understood, which can lead to uncertainties in clinical application. Ethical issues, such as the handling of sensitive genetic information and potential discrimination based on genetic characteristics, require careful regulation and clear data protection guidelines. Access to personalised medicine is also an issue, as advanced genetic tests and therapies are often only available in specialised centres and are financially unaffordable for many patients.

Personalised medicine has the potential to fundamentally change healthcare. By combining genomic information with other data sources, such as lifestyle and environmental factorseven more precise treatment strategies can be developed. Advances in artificial intelligence and big data analysis will further improve the integration and interpretation of this data, which could make personalised medicine more accessible and effective.

Genetic modifications

The social debate on genetic modification is one of the most complex and multi-layered discussions of our time. It encompasses ethical, social, legal and scientific issues arising from the enormous opportunities offered by technologies such as CRISPR-Cas9 and other gene editing tools offer. This debate is fuelled by the rapid development in genome research which is making genetic modifications increasingly accessible and potentially widely applicable. The central themes of this debate concern the opportunities and risks of gene editing, particularly in humans, the impact on society and how the limits of this technology should be defined.

A central topic of the debate is the difference between somatic and germline modifications. Somatic modifications only affect the person being treated and have already been shown to be potentially safe and effective in clinical trials, for example in gene therapy to treat diseases such as sickle cell anaemia. Germline modifications, on the other hand, alter the DNA in eggs, sperm or embryos so that these changes are passed on to future generations. While somatic interventions are widely accepted, germline modifications raise considerable ethical concerns. Critics argue that such interventions are irreversible and could have unintended consequences that only become apparent generations later.

Another aspect is the possibility of creating so-called "designer babies". Gene editing could theoretically be used to promote certain desired traits such as intelligence, physical fitness or even aesthetic characteristics. Such applications raise fundamental questions about the acceptability of genetic optimisation and the impact on social justice. Critics warn of a "genetic divide" where only wealthy sections of society have access to such technologies, which could further exacerbate social inequalities.

The issue of safety also plays a central role. Although technologies such as CRISPR-Cas9 have become more precise, there is still a risk of off-target effects, where unintended genetic changes occur. These could have serious health consequences, especially if they affect germline cells. Such risks emphasise the need for stringent safety and regulatory measures before genetic modifications can be widely applied.

In addition to the technical and ethical issues, genetic modification also raises social and cultural concerns. In many cultures and religious traditions, there are deeply rooted ideas about the sanctity of human life and the role of humans in nature. For some critics, gene editing represents a transgression of moral and natural boundaries that is seen as an interference with creation or divine work. This perspective leads to a broad rejection of the technology, even if it could potentially save lives.

Another important topic is the handling of genetic information and its potential utilisation. Genetic modification requires precise knowledge of the DNA-sequences, which raises the question of data protection and the misuse of such data. There is concern that genetic information could be used for discriminatory practices, for example in the area of insurance or employment. Such scenarios reinforce the call for a clear legal framework and international agreements to ensure the responsible use of the technology.

The global dimension of the debate is also important. While some countries such as the USA, China or the UK research and apply genetic modifications under certain conditions, others have imposed strict bans. This lack of international consensus could lead to a "genetic arms race", with countries competing against each other to dominate advances in gene editing. This raises questions about global justice and co-operation.

However, the positive potential of genetic modification should not be ignored in the debate. Genetic intervention could help millions of people by curing or preventing genetic diseases. The technology could also be used in agriculture to create more resilient plants and secure the global food supply. However, these opportunities require careful consideration of the risks and ethical implications.

2. artificial intelligence

The integration of artificial intelligence (AI) in medicine has enabled far-reaching advances in recent years that are revolutionising diagnosticsrevolutionise diagnostics, therapy and research. AI technologies analyse large amounts of data quickly and precisely, identify patterns and support doctors in their decision-making. Applications such as image analysis in radiology, personalised treatment plans in oncology and AI-supported predictive models in preventive medicine have significantly improved the efficiency and accuracy of medical procedures. By combining big data, machine learning and clinical information, AI opens up new ways to detect diseases earlier, treat them more individually and make healthcare more accessible and effective overall.

Introduction to AI in medicine

Artificial intelligence (AI) has become one of the most influential technologies in medicine in recent years and promises to fundamentally change the way in which diagnoses are made, treatments are carried out and health data is analysed. and analysing health data. AI refers to the use of algorithms and machine learning that can recognise patterns, make predictions and support decisions based on large amounts of data. In medicine, the spectrum of applications ranges from the analysis of medical imaging and the development of personalised therapies to the optimisation of clinical processes and the discovery of new drugs.

The importance of AI in medicine arises from the enormous complexity and wealth of data in modern healthcare. Doctors and researchers are increasingly faced with the challenge of analysing and interpreting large volumes of patient information, genetic data, imaging results and clinical studies. AI offers a solution here by efficiently processing this data and recognising patterns that are barely recognisable to humans. This not only enables faster and more precise diagnoses, but also the identification of individual disease risks and optimised treatment strategies.

A key advantage of AI in medicine is its ability to learn from experience and continuously improve. Algorithms can become increasingly accurate through training with data from clinical practice, contributing to the development of intelligent systems that support, not replace, doctors. This makes AI a tool that enhances the knowledge and skills of professionals while improving the quality and accessibility of healthcare. accessibility of healthcare. However, the introduction of AI into medicine also faces challenges, including ethical issues, data protection and the integration of these technologies into existing systems. Nevertheless, AI is considered one of the most promising approaches to making medicine more efficient, precise and patient-centred.

Relevance of AI in the healthcare sector

The relevance of AI-technologies in healthcare has grown rapidly in recent years and is reflected in their ability to fundamentally improve the efficiency, precision and accessibility of medical care. accessibility of medical care. AI offers solutions to some of the biggest challenges in healthcare, such as processing large amounts of data, making diagnoses more precise and personalising therapies. Machine learning and data analytics can recognise patterns in complex medical data that are difficult for humans to identify, enabling more informed decisions to be made more quickly.

A central area in which AI is is particularly relevant is diagnostics. AI-supported systems, such as those used in radiology or pathology, analyse medical images with high precision and can detect anomalies such as tumours, pneumonia or cardiovascular diseases earlier and more accurately. This leads to better treatment decisions and often to a higher survival rate for patients. In oncology for example, AI models help to analyse the genetic profiles of tumours and suggest targeted treatment options based on a patient's individual genetic characteristics.

AI is also of great importance in preventive medicine is of great importance. Predictive models can be used to recognise individual disease risks at an early stage and suggest preventive measures. Examples include AI systems that predict heart attacks or diabetes risks by combining lifestyle data, genetic information and medical histories.

In addition, AI plays plays a central role in the development of new drugs. Analysing large data sets from genome researchclinical trials and pharmacological databases accelerates the identification of potential active ingredients and significantly reduces the costs of drug development. This became particularly clear during the COVID-19-pandemic, when AI technologies were used to develop potential antiviral agents and vaccine designs more quickly.

AI also improves organisational efficiency in the healthcare sector. Intelligent systems optimise processes in hospitals, for example by predicting patient flows or automating administrative tasks. This frees up medical staff so that they have more time for direct patient care.

Current applications

Artificial intelligence (AI) is increasingly being used in healthcare and has already found a wide range of applications in diagnosticstherapy, prevention and the management of health data revolutionise health data management. One key area of application is medical imaging. AI algorithms analyse X-ray images, CT scans and MRI scans with high precision and support doctors in detecting anomalies such as tumours, pneumonia or cardiovascular diseases. These technologies not only offer faster evaluation, but also greater sensitivity and specificity, especially for subtle findings that are difficult to recognise by the human eye.

Another important area of application is personalised medicine. AI is used to analyse genetic data and other patient-specific information and create personalised treatment plans based on this. In oncology for example, AI models help to identify genetic mutations in tumours that are responsive to specific therapies. This enables targeted treatment that not only increases effectiveness but also reduces side effects. AI is also used in pharmacogenomics to predict how patients will respond to certain drugs, which increases the safety and efficacy of therapies.

In preventive medicine, AI uses predictive models uses predictive models that can predict disease risks. By analysing electronic health records, genetic information and lifestyle data, AI identifies individual risk factors for chronic diseases such as diabetescardiovascular diseases or neurodegenerative diseases. This enables early interventions, such as lifestyle changes or preventive medical measures, which can prevent or delay the onset of disease.

AI also plays a transformative role in drug development also plays a transformative role in drug development. AI algorithms analyse large amounts of data from genomicsclinical studies and chemical libraries to identify and optimise potential active ingredients more quickly. During the COVID-19-pandemic, this technology was used to develop antiviral drugs and vaccine designs more efficiently. AI has significantly accelerated the drug discovery process, reduced costs and improved the chances of success.

AI is also used in the field of robotics and surgical support. is also being utilised. Intelligent surgical systems such as the Da Vinci robot use AI to assist surgeons in minimally invasive procedures by making movements more precise and minimising risks. These technologies help to reduce patient recovery time and increase the success rates of surgical procedures.

Another relevant area of application for AI is the management and analysis of large volumes of medical data. Electronic health records are optimised by AI by automatically classifying data, reducing errors and providing information for clinical decisions. Intelligent systems help to integrate patient data from different sources, providing a comprehensive overview of a patient's state of health.

In infection control, AI is used to is used to predict and monitor disease outbreaks. For example, by analysing epidemiological data and travel data, AI was able to help model the spread of the virus during the COVID-19-pandemic, AI helped to model the spread of the virus and identify hotspots at an early stage. This has helped governments and healthcare systems to plan preventive measures more effectively.

AI is also used in mental health application. Chatbots and virtual assistants based on AI offer support in the treatment of depressionanxiety disorders and other mental illnesses. These systems can recognise symptoms, provide individual support and refer patients to therapists if necessary. AI-supported apps are also used to analyse behavioural data and provide personalised recommendations to improve mental health.

Overall, AI enables in healthcare enables more precise diagnoses, more individualised therapies, more effective prevention strategies and more efficient workflows. It has the potential to improve the quality of patient care and reduce healthcare costs at the same time. Despite these advances, challenges such as ensuring data protectiondata protection, the avoidance of algorithmic bias and the ethical use of the technology. However, as development and integration progresses, AI will play an even more central role in the future of healthcare.

AI in medical imaging

The use of artificial intelligence (AI) in medical imaging has made considerable progress in recent years and is revolutionising fields such as radiology and pathology. AI technologies, in particular machine learning and deep learning, analyse large amounts of complex image data with an accuracy and speed that surpasses conventional methods. These applications enable more precise diagnosticsimprove the efficiency of workflows and support doctors in their decision-making.

In radiology, AI is is often used to analyse X-ray, CT and MRI images. Algorithms can reliably identify anomalies such as tumours, fractures, bleeding or pneumonia. In oncology in particular AI has shown that it can detect small, difficult-to-detect tumours at an early stage, which significantly increases patients' chances of survival. One example is the use of AI in the detection of lung cancer on CT scans, where algorithms can precisely localise suspicious nodules and reduce the risk of misinterpretation.

In pathology, AI is used is used to analyse digital tissue samples (digital pathology). Deep learning models recognise cellular patterns and morphological changes that are indicative of diseases such as cancer diseases such as cancer, often faster and more accurately than human pathologists. AI systems can identify specific genetic and molecular markers in tissue samples that are crucial for the choice of therapy. These technologies not only speed up diagnosticsbut also support the personalisation of treatments.

A particular advantage of AI in medical imaging is its ability to analyse large image databases and learn from millions of cases. This allows algorithms to be continuously optimised to improve their accuracy and reliability. AI-supported tools such as computer-aided detection (CAD) systems are increasingly being used in clinical practice to support radiologists in reporting, particularly in mammography for the early detection of breast cancer or in the analysis of CT scans for the assessment of COVID-19-related lung damage.

In addition to improving diagnostic precision, AI also optimises also optimises efficiency in radiology and pathology. Automated systems reduce the time needed for image analysis and relieve doctors of routine tasks, allowing them to focus on more complex cases and patient-centred activities. At the same time, AI can serve as quality assurance by providing a second opinion on findings and minimising human error.

Despite these advances, there are challenges when it comes to integrating AI into medical imaging. One of the biggest is ensuring data security and privacy, as AI systems need to be trained on large amounts of sensitive patient data. In addition, validation of the algorithms in clinical practice is essential to ensure that they function robustly and reliably. Another important aspect is acceptance by medical staff, as doctors often have reservations about fully trusting AI systems, especially when making critical decisions.

AI-supported therapy planning

AI-assisted decision-making and treatment planning has the potential to fundamentally change medical care by enabling more accurate diagnoses and more personalised treatment approaches. AI systems use complex algorithms and machine learning to analyse large amounts of medical data - including patient history, genetic profiles, imaging and clinical trials - and derive recommendations. These technologies support doctors in choosing optimal therapies and help to make treatment decisions faster, more informed and more personalised.

A key area of application is oncologywhere AI-models are used to analyse genetic and molecular data from tumours. These analyses identify specific mutations or biomarkers that respond to certain therapies, such as targeted drugs or immunotherapies. By integrating data from clinical trials, AI systems can also make suggestions for experimental therapies or participation in trials that may be relevant for the patient in question. This not only increases the effectiveness of treatment, but also opens up new options for patients with complex or rare types of cancer.

In pharmacogenomics AI is used is used to predict how a patient will react to certain drugs. This is particularly relevant when choosing the dosage or drug to minimise side effects and maximise efficacy. For example, AI systems can suggest alternative drugs or customise dosages for patients with genetic variants that affect their ability to metabolise drugs. These personalised approaches help to reduce the risk of treatment failure or adverse effects.

Another example is AI-supported therapy planning for chronic diseases such as diabetes or cardiovascular diseases. Here, algorithms can analyse patient data such as blood pressure, blood sugar levels, lifestyle and previous treatments to create tailored treatment plans. These plans can include both pharmacological and non-pharmacological interventions, such as dietary changes or exercise therapies that are specifically tailored to the patient's individual needs.

In intensive care medicine, too AI is playing is also playing a growing role. Algorithms continuously analyse patients' vital data and detect changes that could indicate a deterioration in their condition at an early stage. These early warning systems can make suggestions for interventions, such as adjusting medication dosages, ventilation parameters or fluid intake to prevent complications.

One area in which AI-supported decision making is also showing great progress is rehabilitation. Here, AI systems can monitor the course of therapy and suggest individually optimised rehabilitation plans based on progress data. This dynamic adaptation enables more efficient recovery and a higher quality of life for patients.

Improved diagnostics and increased efficiency

The integration of AI in medicine has fundamentally improved fundamentally improved diagnostics and significantly increased the efficiency of clinical processes. AI algorithms, especially those based on machine learning and deep learning, are able to analyse large amounts of medical data, such as imaging, genetic information and patient records, with a speed and precision that far exceeds human capabilities. These capabilities make AI an indispensable tool in modern medicine.

In diagnostics AI enables enables more precise detection of diseases, often at very early stages. In radiology, for example, AI-supported systems can analyse CT scans, MRIs and X-ray images and identify anomalies such as tumours, fractures or inflammatory changes, often with an accuracy that matches or even exceeds that of human experts. Especially for hard-to-detect findings, such as early tumours or subtle lung abnormalities, AI has shown to provide higher sensitivity and specificity through its ability to detect subtle patterns. This leads to earlier diagnoses and enables timely treatment, which can significantly improve the prognosis for patients.

AI also plays a transformative role in pathology is also playing a transformative role. By analysing digitised tissue samples, AI can identify cellular changes that indicate diseases such as cancer. diseases such as cancer. Algorithms can not only recognise tumour tissue, but also analyse the molecular signature of a tumour, which is crucial for the selection of targeted therapies. These technologies save time and reduce the risk of diagnostic errors by providing standardised and reproducible results.

In addition to improved diagnostics AI contributes makes a significant contribution to increasing efficiency in clinical processes. Routine tasks such as analysing image data, screening patient of patient records or the coding of medical information can be automated, reducing the workload for doctors and medical staff. This creates more time for direct patient care and reduces the burden of administrative tasks. One example is the automation of screening programmes, for example in mammographywhere AI systems prioritise suspicious findings and thus reduce the radiologists' workload.

AI can also act as a quality assurance tool by reviewing human diagnoses and highlighting potential errors or missed findings. This function is particularly valuable in busy clinics or in regions with limited access to specialised doctors. At the same time, AI can increase the consistency and accuracy of diagnostic processes, which in turn improves the reliability of medical care.

Another area in which AI increases efficiency is the optimisation of clinical processes. Predictive models can analyse the flow of patients in hospitals and predict which resources will be needed in the coming days or weeks. This information helps to optimise the use of beds, staff and medical equipment and avoid bottlenecks. AI systems can also help to make ordering medication or scheduling appointments more efficient.

Bias and interpretability of AI-models

The challenges with regard to bias and the interpretability of AI models are key obstacles to the integration of AI technologies into medicine.-models are key obstacles to the integration of AI technologies into medicine. These two aspects are closely linked and concern both the technical development and the ethical and clinical implications of the use of AI in healthcare.

Bias in AI-models occurs when the algorithms deliver incorrect or unfair results due to insufficient or distorted training data. In medicine, this can have serious consequences, as decisions about diagnoses, treatment recommendations or resource allocations directly affect the health and well-being of patients. For example, an AI system that has been trained on data that predominantly comes from a specific population group can deliver inaccurate or unfavourable results for patients of other ethnicities or genders. A well-known example is the underrepresentation of women or ethnic minorities in clinical trials, which can lead to lower accuracy of models in these groups. This reinforces existing inequalities in healthcare and jeopardises the equity and reliability of care.

Another factor for bias is the quality of the training data. Medical data can be incorrect, incomplete or influenced by systematic biases, which are then transferred to the results of the AI. results. For example, biases contained in electronic health records, such as inconsistent diagnoses or treatment decisions in the past, can negatively influence the performance of an AI system. These biases can be unintentionally perpetuated or even amplified if they are not recognised and addressed early on.

The interpretability of AI-models is another major challenge, especially in medicine, where life and death decisions are made. Many modern AI algorithms, especially deep learning models, are often designed as "black boxes" where the internal decision-making processes are difficult to understand. This lack of transparency can affect healthcare professionals' trust in AI systems and hinder their acceptance. Doctors and patients must be able to understand how and why an AI system arrives at a particular diagnosis or recommendation in order to make informed decisions. Without this traceability, the responsibility for medical for medical decisions remains unclear, which raises ethical and legal questions.

The lack of interpretability also has practical consequences. If an AI-model makes a misdiagnosis or makes an incorrect treatment recommendation, for example, it is difficult to identify the source of the error and rectify it. This not only makes it more difficult to improve the models, but can also make them less effective and trustworthy.

Overcoming these challenges requires a multidisciplinary approach. To reduce bias, representative and high quality data reflecting the diversity of patient groups must be used. This requires investment in data collection and the promotion of inclusive clinical trials. In addition, technical approaches such as bias correction algorithms or adversarial training can be used to recognise and reduce bias in the data.

Approaches such as Explainable AI (XAI), which aim to make the decision-making processes of models understandable and transparent, are promising for improving interpretability. Visualisations, feature analyses and rule-based algorithms can help to better explain the logic behind the recommendations of an AI system.-system's recommendations better. At the same time, regulatory frameworks must be created that promote transparency and accountability.

Responsibility

The responsibility for AI-based decisions in the medical context raises a variety of ethical, legal and practical issues that require particular attention in a highly sensitive area such as healthcare. As AI is increasingly used in diagnostic and therapeutic processes, clear responsibilities need to be defined to ensure trust in these technologies and that they are used for the benefit of patients. Ethical aspects and data protection play a central role here.

The integration of AI into medical practice is leading to a shift in responsibilities, particularly in relation to decision-making. While doctors are traditionally responsible for diagnoses and treatment decisions, AI systems can significantly influence these processes through their ability to analyse complex data and make recommendations. Nevertheless, the question remains as to who is ultimately responsible if an AI system makes a misdiagnosis or recommends an inappropriate therapy. Is it the developer of the AI, the operator of the technology, the medical staff or the institution using the AI?

Current ethical practice is for doctors to retain the final decision-making authority and to critically review the recommendations of the AI. critically review the AI's recommendations. However, this presupposes that they understand how the AI works and can interpret its results, which is not always the case with highly complex models such as deep learning. This gives rise to an ethical responsibilityto design AI systems in such a way that they are explainable (Explainable AI, XAI) and comprehensible for medical staff. Otherwise, there is a risk of an "automation trap" in which doctors blindly rely on AI without critically scrutinising its recommendations.

From an ethical perspective, the use of AI should should always be patient-centred. This means that the benefit for patients must be the top priority, without jeopardising their dignity, rights or safety. A key aspect is fairness. AI systems must not contain systematic biases that penalise certain population groups. This requires representative training data and mechanisms for recognising and correcting bias.

Another ethical issue is transparency. Patients and medical staff have a right to know how AI systems arrive at their decisions.-systems arrive at their decisions. The lack of interpretability of many AI models poses a challenge here, as patients may not be able to understand why a certain diagnosis was made or a therapy suggested. This could lead to a loss of trust in the technology.

Informed consent also plays an important role. Patients must be informed that AI will be used in their diagnostic or therapeutic process and they should have the opportunity to decide in favour of or against its use. This requires clear communication and an understandable presentation of the function and potential limitations of AI.

Data protection is another sensitive aspect in the medical context, as AI systems are-systems are trained on large amounts of personal and often highly sensitive data. The processing of this data must comply with strict data protection laws such as the General Data Protection Regulation (GDPR) in the EU. Patients must be informed about how their data is collected, stored and used, and their consent must be obtained.

3. immunotherapy

Immunotherapy has established itself in modern medicine as a revolutionary approach that utilises the body's own immune system to combat diseases, especially cancer.to fight diseases, especially cancer. Through targeted strategies such as checkpoint inhibitorsCAR-T cell therapies and monoclonal antibodies the immune system is activated or modulated to recognise and destroy tumour cells more effectively. These advances have significantly expanded the treatment options and open up new perspectives for the treatment of cancer, autoimmune diseases and chronic infections. and chronic infections.

Scientific foundations

Modern immunotherapies are based on the targeted modulation of the immune system in order to treat diseases such as cancerautoimmune diseases and chronic infections more effectively. The scientific basis lies in a deep understanding of how the immune system works, in particular the mechanisms by which it distinguishes between the body's own cells and pathogens or abnormal cells such as tumours. The core principle is the ability of the immune system to recognise and react to specific antigens, with T cells and B cells play a central role.

A key concept of immunotherapy is the overcoming of immune checkpoint mechanisms. These checkpoints, such as CTLA-4 and PD-1/PD-L1, regulate the activity of T cells and prevent excessive immune reactions. and prevent excessive immune reactions. Tumour cells often use these mechanisms to evade immune recognition. Checkpoint inhibitorssuch as monoclonal antibodies against PD-1 or CTLA-4, block these signalling pathways and reactivate the immune response against the tumour.

Another foundation of immunotherapy is the development of CAR T cell therapiesin which a patient's T cells of a patient are genetically modified so that they recognise specific tumour antigens and attack them in a targeted manner. These personalised cell therapies have shown remarkable success, particularly in haematological cancers.

The use of monoclonal antibodies that specifically target tumour antigens or stimulate the immune system is another pillar of immunotherapy. These antibodies selectively bind to cancer cells and mark them for destruction by the immune system.

The scientific advances in immunotherapy are based on a combination of findings from immunologymolecular biology and genetics. These disciplines have contributed to a better understanding of the interactions between immune cells, tumours and the microenvironment and to the development of therapeutic approaches based on this knowledge, which are fundamentally changing medicine.

How immunotherapy works

Immunotherapy uses the body's own immune system to treat diseases such as cancerinfections or autoimmune diseases by activating, strengthening or specifically modulating its natural defence mechanisms. Its mode of operation is based on the immune system's ability to differentiate between the body's own cells and foreign or abnormal cells and to combat these in a targeted manner.

A central mechanism is the activation or modulation of T cellsa crucial component of adaptive immunity. T cells use specific receptors to recognise antigens that are presented on the surface of target cells. However, tumour cells or infected cells can develop mechanisms to evade immune recognition by expressing immunoregulatory molecules such as PD-L1, which inhibit the activity of T cells. Checkpoint inhibitorsa form of immunotherapyblock such inhibitory signals (e.g. through antibodies against PD-1 or against PD-1 or CTLA-4) and reactivate the T-cell response against the tumour.

Another approach, CAR T-cell therapy, involves the genetic modification of T-cellsso that they can recognise and destroy specific tumour antigens. This personalised therapy is used in particular for haematological cancers such as leukaemia.

Monoclonal antibodies are another important strategy in immunotherapy. They bind specifically to antigens on the surface of tumour cells, mark them for destruction by immune cells or block signalling pathways that promote tumour growth. Some antibodies can also have immunostimulatory effects by activating immune cells.

In addition, other immunotherapies utilise substances such as cytokines (e.g. interleukin-2 or interferons), which promote the growth and activity of immune cells. Vaccines that prepare the immune system for tumour or viral antigens are also part of immunotherapy.

Overall, immunotherapy works works by specifically enhancing, redirecting or reactivating the natural immune response to combat pathological cells that have previously evaded immune surveillance. The combination of these approaches opens up new possibilities for the treatment of serious diseases and has significantly expanded the therapeutic spectrum of modern medicine.

Applications in oncology

Checkpoint inhibitorssuch as PD-1/PD-L1 inhibitors, are an innovative form of immunotherapythat reactivate the immune system to fight tumour cells more effectively. They target so-called immune checkpoints, which act as natural brakes on the immune system to prevent excessive immune reactions and autoimmune diseases. prevent autoimmune diseases. However, tumour cells use these mechanisms to evade immune surveillance and inhibit the activity of T cellsthat would normally attack tumour cells.

The PD-1/PD-L1 pathway plays a central role in this process. **PD-1 (Programmed Death-1)** is a receptor on the surface of T cellsthat is activated when it binds to its ligand **PD-L1 (programmed death ligand 1)** or PD-L2, which can be expressed on tumour cells or other immune cells. Activation of this signalling pathway leads to inhibition of T-cell activity and thus to a dampening of the immune response. Tumour cells that express PD-L1 in high concentrations use this mechanism to "switch off" T cells and avoid destruction by the immune system.

Checkpoint inhibitors are monoclonal antibodiesthat block either PD-1 or PD-L1 and thus interrupt the inhibitory signalling pathway. This blockade keeps the T cell active and allows it to attack the tumour cells. This effect reactivates the immune response and enables the immune system to eliminate tumour cells that have previously evaded immune recognition.

The clinical efficacy of PD-1/PD-L1 inhibitors has led to their use in the treatment of various types of cancer, including melanoma, non-small cell lung cancer (NSCLC), bladder cancer and renal cell carcinoma. Examples of approved PD-1 inhibitors **include nivolumab** and **pembrolizumab**, while **atezolizumab** and **durvalumab** are well-known PD-L1 inhibitors.

Checkpoint inhibitorscheckpoint inhibitors, particularly PD-1 and PD-L1 inhibitors, are ground-breaking immunotherapies that aim to reactivate the body's own immune system to fight tumour cells. They block so-called immune checkpoints that tumour cells use to evade immune surveillance. These checkpoints normally regulate the activity of T-cells and prevent excessive immune reactions, but are exploited by tumour cells to suppress an immune response.

PD-1 (Programmed Death-1) is a receptor that is expressed on activated T cells. cells. When it binds to its ligand PD-L1 (programmed death ligand 1), which can occur on tumour cells or immunoregulatory cells in the tumour microenvironment, the activity of the T cells is inhibited. This interaction protects the tumour cells from destruction by the immune system.

Checkpoint inhibitors such as PD-1 inhibitors (**pembrolizumab, nivolumab**) or PD-L1 inhibitors (**atezolizumab, durvalumab**) interrupt this signalling pathway by blocking either the PD-1 receptor on T cells or the PD-L1 ligand on tumour cells. The blockade maintains T-cell activity and reactivates the immune response against tumour cells. The T cells can now recognise and destroy tumour cells.

This mode of action has revolutionised the treatment of cancer especially for tumours such as melanoma, non-small cell lung cancer (NSCLC), renal cell carcinoma and bladder cancer. Efficacy often depends on the expression of PD-L1 on tumour cells, which can be used as a biomarker for treatment decisions.

CAR T-cell therapy (Chimeric Antigen Receptor T-Cell Therapy) is a highly innovative form of immunotherapy that uses genetically modified T-cells.that uses genetically modified T-cells cells to specifically target cancer cells. This approach has achieved remarkable clinical success in recent years, particularly in haematological cancers such as acute lymphoblastic leukaemia (ALL) and certain forms of B-cell lymphoma.

The therapy is based on genetically modifying the patient's T cells of the patient in such a way that they are equipped with a chimeric antigen receptor (CAR). This receptor combines the antigen-binding ability of an antibody with the activation ability of T cells. The CAR is designed to recognise specific antigens on the surface of tumour cells, e.g. CD19, a marker that is frequently expressed in B-cell malignancies. The modified T cells are infused into the patient, where they specifically attack and destroy the tumour cells.

The clinical success of CAR-T cell therapy is impressive. In the treatment of ALL in children and young adults who do not respond to conventional therapies, CAR-T cells have shown remission rates of up to 80 %. have shown remission rates of up to 80 %. Similarly remarkable results have been achieved in patients with relapsed or refractory B-cell lymphomas. Products such as **tisagenlecleucel** (Kymriah) and **axicabtagene-ciloleucel** (Yescarta) are already approved and have been shown to be highly effective, even in patients with limited treatment options.

Despite these successes, there are challenges. The production of CAR-T cells is complex, time-consuming and expensive, as it has to be customised for each individual patient. In addition, side effects such as cytokine release syndrome (CRS) and neurological toxicities are common, although usually treatable. These complications require close monitoring and specific interventions.

CAR-T cell therapy has revolutionised the treatment of haematological cancers and is inspiring further research to extend its application to solid tumours. Despite existing challenges, it shows the potential to lead immunotherapy into a new era where personalised and targeted approaches can significantly improve treatment outcomes.

Use for autoimmune diseases

The use of immunotherapy for autoimmune diseases has gained considerable importance in recent years, as these approaches can specifically intervene in the dysregulated mechanisms of the immune system. Autoimmune diseases such as rheumatoid arthritis, systemic lupus erythematosus (SLE), multiple sclerosis (MS) or Crohn's disease are caused by an overactive or misdirected immune response in which the immune system attacks the body's own tissues. Immunotherapies aim to modulate these dysregulated processes and restore the balance of the immune system.

A key approach is the use of monoclonal antibodies that specifically block signalling pathways or molecules that are responsible for the excessive immune response. Examples include **TNF-alpha inhibitors** such as infliximab or adalimumab, which inhibit the activity of tumour necrosis factor alpha (TNF-α), a key mediator of inflammation in inflammatory diseases such as rheumatoid arthritis and Crohn's disease. **IL-6 inhibitors** (e.g. tocilizumab) also block inflammatory signalling pathways that are overactive in autoimmune diseases. are overactive in autoimmune diseases.

Checkpoint inhibitorswhich were originally developed for cancer immunotherapy, are also being researched to modulate the activity of certain immune cells in autoimmune diseases. diseases. They can help to restore the immune system's self-tolerance by strengthening regulatory T cells or dampening excessive immune reactions. or dampening excessive immune reactions.

Another innovative approach is **B-cell depletion**, in which B-cells that produce antibodies against the body's own tissue are specifically eliminated. Rituximab, an antibody against CD20, is used successfully in SLE and rheumatoid arthritis.

Future strategies include cell therapies in which regulatory T cells (Tregs) are modified and (Tregs) are modified and multiplied ex vivo to specifically suppress autoimmunity in the body. These personalised approaches could enable long-term remissions and reduce the side effects of conventional therapies.

Immunotherapy for autoimmune diseases has revolutionised the treatment landscape by offering more specific, more effective and often better tolerated alternatives to conventional immunosuppressants. By combining targeted therapies and personalised approaches, these therapies are expected to become even more widely used in the future and significantly improve patients' quality of life.

Treatment of chronic infections

The treatment of chronic infections poses a particular challenge, as pathogens such as viruses, bacteria or parasites often evade the defence mechanisms of the immune system and drug therapy. Chronic infections such as HIVhepatitis B (HBV), hepatitis C (HCV), tuberculosis and herpes viruses can persist by forming latent reservoirs that prevent complete eradication. Advances in immunotherapy and drug research offer innovative approaches to combat these infections more effectively.

One of the key strategies is to strengthen the immune response to enable the body to better control or eliminate the pathogen. Immunotherapeutic approaches such as **checkpoint inhibitors** are being researched to reactivate the T-cell response against chronic viral infections such as HIV and HBV. These mechanisms are of interest because chronic infections often cause immune exhaustion (T-cell exhaustion), which impairs the immune system's ability to fight the pathogen.

Another innovative approach is **therapeutic vaccination**, in which specific vaccines boost the immune response against persistent pathogens. In contrast to prophylactic vaccines, therapeutic vaccines aim to help people who are already infected by stimulating the immune system to control or reduce viral reservoirs. This strategy is being intensively researched for HIV and HBV in particular.

Antiviral drugs, such as direct-acting antivirals (DAAs), have proven to be effective in the treatment of chronic infections such as hepatitis C have made enormous progress. DAAs target specific viral proteins that are essential for the replication of the virus and have achieved cure rates of over 95%. Similarly successful are combination therapies for HIVwhich consist of antiretroviral drugs that block various steps of the viral life cycle. These treatments are highly effective but require lifelong use as they only suppress the viral load but do not eliminate the reservoirs.

For chronic bacterial infections such as tuberculosis intensive research is being conducted into immunomodulators that can activate the immune system and at the same time overcome antibiotic resistance. antibiotic resistance. New vaccines are also being developed that not only prevent the infection but could also have a therapeutic effect.

Future approaches include the combination of immunotherapies with gene therapiesto eliminate latent infections such as HIV targeted elimination. Technologies such as CRISPR-Cas9 are being researched to remove viral genomes genomes directly from infected cells, which could potentially enable a cure.

The treatment of chronic infections benefits from an increasing combination of immunologymolecular biology and modern therapy methods. While the complete cure of many chronic infections remains a challenge, advances in immunotherapy and targeted drug development promise significant improvements for patients. and targeted drug development promise significant improvements for patients.

4. comparison and synthesis of progress

Similarities

The various approaches of modern immunotherapies and gene therapies - such as CAR-T cell therapiescheckpoint inhibitors and therapeutic vaccines - all contribute to the development of personalised medicine. They are based on a deep understanding of individual biological characteristics, be it the genetic make-up of the patient, the specific properties of tumours or the molecular mechanisms of a disease. These therapies enable customised treatment strategies that are specifically tailored to the individual needs of a patient. Through the integration of genomicsproteomics and immunology they address the specific causes of diseases and improve the precision and effectiveness of treatment.

Differences

In terms of **clinical implementation and accessibility** these approaches differ considerably. Checkpoint inhibitors such as PD-1/PD-L1 inhibitors are standardised drugs that can be administered relatively easily and are available in many clinical settings. CAR-T cell therapies on the other hand, require specialised treatment centres and individual adaptation for each patient. Therapeutic vaccines fall between these extremes and are often tailored to specific target populations.

The **costs and infrastructure requirements** also vary greatly. Checkpoint inhibitors are comparatively cheaper and more easily scalable due to standardised production. CAR-T cell therapies on the other hand, are very expensive as they are produced on a patient-specific basis and require complex processes such as cell collection, modification and reinfusion. Therapeutic vaccines can also incur considerable costs depending on the production method and target group, but are often easier to implement.

Assessment of relevance

The relevance of these approaches is undisputed, as they open up new possibilities for the treatment of difficult-to-treat diseases. CAR-T cell therapies are particularly ground-breaking in haematological cancers, while checkpoint inhibitors have achieved impressive results in solid tumours and metastatic diseases. Therapeutic vaccines could be used both preventively and curatively in broad patient populations. However, the choice of the best option depends on the specific disease, availability and individual patient needs.

Production, logistics and scalability

The production of modern therapies such as CAR-T cells is indeed a demanding and complex process that poses numerous challenges. These patient-specific therapies require a high degree of precision and customisation, as the cells of each individual patient must be genetically modified ex vivo and then reinfused. The associated just-in-time production, in which each treatment is customised, poses considerable logistical challenges.

The manufacturing process begins with the collection of T cells from the patient by leukapheresis. These cells are genetically modified in specialised laboratories under sterile conditions so that they express a chimeric antigen receptor (CAR) that specifically recognises tumour cells. The cells are then expanded, quality-checked and prepared for return to the patient. Each of these steps is technically demanding and must be carried out under strictly controlled conditions to ensure the safety and efficacy of the therapy.

The patient-specific nature of CAR-T cell therapy poses considerable logistical difficulties. As the cells can only be used by the patient in question, collection, modification and reinfusion must be closely coordinated to avoid delays or contamination. The entire process is time-critical, as the cells must be transported and processed within a narrow time window. This is particularly challenging for global distribution, as the cells often have to be transported over long distances, for example from a collection centre in one country to a specialised laboratory in another.

The production of CAR-T cells is currently only scalable to a limited extent, as it is highly customised and labour-intensive. The availability of specialised production facilities and qualified specialists is far from sufficient to meet the increasing demand. This not only leads to longer waiting times for patients, but also significantly increases costs. The development of automated and standardised production processes could provide a remedy here, but is still in the development phase.

CAR-T cells are extremely sensitive to external influences such as temperature and time. They must be transported in cryogenic or controlled environments in order to maintain their viability and functionality. The smallest errors in storage or logistics can render the therapy ineffective. The infrastructure for such specialised transport is expensive and limited in many regions.

Research institutions and companies are working on various approaches to overcome these challenges. Automated manufacturing processes could simplify and speed up production, while advances in cell storage and transport technology could help to improve the robustness of the cells. Decentralised production models, in which cell processing centres are located closer to the patients, could simplify logistics and shorten transport times.

Ethical aspects

The ethical challenges are manifold and include the accessibilityequity and possible long-term consequences of the therapies. High costs may limit availability and increase health inequalities, as only wealthier countries or population groups may have access to these innovative therapies. The genetic modification of cells, particularly in the germline, raises questions about possible undesirable consequences for future generations. There is also a risk that the focus on expensive, highly specialised therapies will result in fewer resources being made available for more widely applicable approaches. Data protection is also a key issue, as many of these therapies require extensive genetic and medical data that must be protected from misuse.

6. social implications

Social impact of new therapies

The introduction of modern therapies such as CAR-T cellscheckpoint inhibitors and gene therapies has far-reaching social implications. They offer revolutionary possibilities for the treatment of serious diseases, but raise fundamental questions regarding accessibilityequity, data protection and the responsibility of the actors involved.

Accessibility and justice

The unequal distribution of modern therapies is one of the most pressing problems. These innovative approaches are often associated with extremely high costs, which limits their access to wealthier regions and social classes. Countries with limited resources often do not have the necessary infrastructure, qualified personnel or funding to offer such treatments. Even in wealthy countries, access is often limited to patients covered by private insurance or special programmes.

This inequality increases the discrepancy in global healthcare and leads to ethical questions: who decides who gets access to these life-saving therapies and how can they be distributed fairly? Models such as subsidised pricing models, international partnerships or nonprofit programmes could help to promote equity, but are still insufficiently established.

The introduction of new technologies also requires considerable investment in infrastructure, research and development. Regions with advanced medical technology benefit directly, while developing countries are often excluded. Social and economic differences within a country can also have a significant impact on access. Patients in rural areas often have less access to specialised treatment centres, which are necessary for the implementation of modern therapies.

The global distribution of such technologies therefore requires international cooperation. Strategies such as technology transfer, training of specialists and investment in local production capacities could help to close the gap between different regions. At the same time, pricing models must be developed to make the therapies affordable for low-income countries.

Data protection and privacy

Modern therapies are often based on the analysis of sensitive genetic and medical data. This raises considerable data protection issues. The storage, processing and use of this data harbours risks such as unauthorised access, data leaks or misuse, for example by insurance companies or employers. The risk of sensitive information being misused is particularly high in countries with weak data protection laws.

Responsibility and regulation

The responsibility for the development, distribution and safe use of modern therapies lies with a variety of stakeholders, including research institutions, companies, governments and international organisations. Research organisations and industry have a responsibility to make technologies safe, effective and affordable. At the same time, they must act transparently and commit to ethical standards.

Governments play a key role in regulating these therapies to ensure their safety and efficacy. They must also ensure that the therapies are fairly distributed and made accessible. Subsidies, tax breaks and government-funded programmes could help to make the therapies more widely available.

International organisations such as the WHO are crucial to setting global standards for safety, ethics and justice. and justice. They can also act as intermediaries between wealthy and low-income countries to improve access to life-saving therapies. They should also develop mechanisms that facilitate technology transfer and support countries with limited resources.

7. outlook

The future of medicine is increasingly being shaped by synergies between genomicsartificial intelligence (AI) and immunotherapy will be characterised by synergies. These disciplines complement each other and have the potential to improve diagnosticsprevention and therapy to a completely new level. While genomics enables a deep understanding of the genetic basis of health and disease, AI uses this data to recognise patterns, make predictions and optimise treatment strategies. Immunotherapies complement this spectrum by creating targeted treatment approaches that activate or modify the body's natural defence mechanisms.

Synergies between genomics, AI and immunotherapy

The integration of these technologies offers immense opportunities. Genomic analyses identify specific genetic variations or mutations that can serve as targets for immunotherapies, while AI-algorithms accelerate the analysis of this data and recognise patterns that are crucial for therapy planning. AI can also support the development of new immunotherapies by analysing large amounts of data from clinical trials, molecular research and real patient data. The combination of AI and genomics potential target structures for CAR-T cell therapies or checkpoint or checkpoint inhibitors faster and more precisely, which shortens the time to clinical application.

Research gaps

Despite impressive progress, there are still numerous unanswered questions and areas of research. One of the key challenges is to improve the efficacy of immunotherapies for solid tumours, as these are often less responsive than haematological cancers. The complex interaction between tumours, the immune response and the microenvironment is not yet fully understood. In addition, the long-term effects of immunotherapies and gene therapiesespecially in the case of germline modificationsremain unclear.

Another field of research is the integration and standardisation of data from different sources, such as genomicsepigenetics and proteomicsto create more comprehensive models for precision medicine. There is also a lack of large-scale studies investigating the effectiveness and safety of new approaches in diverse populations to avoid health inequalities. Furthermore, there are still no established methods to reduce costs while ensuring the quality of therapies.

Identification of further fields of application

The technologies have the potential to go beyond their previous areas of application. In infectiology personalised vaccines and immunotherapies could help combat chronic or novel infections such as HIV or resistant tuberculosiscould revolutionise the fight against chronic or novel infections. In autoimmunity, there are opportunities to specifically modify regulatory T cells cells in order to dampen misdirected immune reactions. In preventive medicine, too, genomic and AI-based approaches could also help to recognise disease risks at an early stage and adapt preventive measures to individual patients.

Implications for medical practice

The integration of genomics, AI and immunotherapy will fundamentally change medical practice. Doctors will increasingly have to deal with complex technologies and be able to interpret the results of AI-supported analyses and genomic tests. This requires continuous training and interdisciplinary collaboration between doctors, bioinformaticians and engineers.

Patients could take an increasingly active role in their healthcare by accessing personalised information about genetic risks and treatment options. This will change the way patients interact with doctors and make decisions. At the same time, healthcare is becoming increasingly data-driven, with electronic health records, genomic databases and AIsupported systems will be key components of clinical decision-making.

Long-term changes in the healthcare sector due to new technologies

The long-term changes in the healthcare system brought about by these technologies are significant. The healthcare system will move from reactive disease treatment to preventive, patient-centred and data-based care. Genomic and AI-based diagnostics will make it possible to detect diseases earlier, before symptoms appear, and to customise preventive measures. Therapies will be increasingly customised, which will increase effectiveness and minimise side effects.

At the same time, the cost structures in the healthcare sector are being redefined. Although the initial investment in these technologies is high, long-term savings could be realised through more precise diagnoses, targeted therapies and the reduction of ineffective treatments. Nevertheless, challenges remain in terms of accessibility and equity remain, which need to be addressed through policy measures, international co-operation and technological innovation.

8. conclusion

This presentation of the major medical advances of recent years impressively demonstrates how far-reaching and diverse the achievements of modern medicine have been during this period. They bear witness not only to the enormous innovative power and creativity in research, but also to the ability to efficiently translate theoretical findings into clinical practice in order to significantly improve the lives of patients worldwide.

One of the key aspects of recent developments is the increasing individualisation of medical approaches. Advances in personalised medicine, particularly in oncology, make it possible to tailor treatments to the genetic and molecular characteristics of each individual patient. This has not only increased cancer survival rates, but also significantly reduced side effects and the burden on patients. At the same time, technologies such as CRISPR-Cas have revolutionised gene therapy by enabling precise interventions in the genome. They therefore offer new prospects for curing previously incurable genetic diseases.

The digitalisation of healthcare and the integration of artificial intelligence represent another milestone. AI-powered algorithms can analyse vast amounts of data to identify complex patterns that are difficult for humans to access. This has significantly increased diagnostic accuracy, particularly in radiology and pathology, while also providing doctors with valuable support in making treatment planning decisions. Digitalisation has also improved telemedicine and patient data management, enabling more efficient care, especially in remote or underserved regions.

Advances in surgical techniques, particularly the development of minimally invasive procedures, also deserve special recognition. These techniques significantly reduce the burden on patients, enable shorter hospital stays and minimise post-operative complications. Together with innovations in organ transplantation, such as machine perfusion for the preservation of donor organs, these developments have raised the treatment options in surgery and transplantation medicine to a new level.

The groundbreaking successes in vaccine development, particularly in connection with the COVID-19 pandemic, should also be emphasised. The rapid development and availability of mRNA vaccines illustrate how powerful modern biomedical research can be when science, technology and international collaboration work seamlessly together. These successes impressively demonstrate how crucial the promotion and funding of medical research is for overcoming global health crises.

10. index

Adenine 35
Alzheimer's 20, 32, 49
Amniocentesis 42
Anxiety disorders 62
Antibiotics 11, 21
Antibiotic resistance 89
Antibodies 78, 80, 87
Autoimmune diseases 77, 79, 81, 86, 87
Biotechnology 18, 22, 24
Breast cancer 39, 47, 64
CAR-T cell therapies 77, 78, 91, 92, 102
Checkpoint inhibitors 77, 78, 80, 81, 82, 83, 87, 88, 91, 92, 97, 102
Chemotherapies 12, 47
chronic infections 88, 89, 90
Clopidogrel 48
COVID-19 15, 36, 41, 58, 61, 64
CRISPR-Cas9 13, 23, 25, 30, 31, 32, 33, 44, 50, 52, 90
Cytosine 35

Data protection 30, 53, 57, 62, 73, 75, 95, 97, 99
Depression 62
Diabetes 12, 15, 26, 32, 49, 60, 67
Diagnostics 11, 12, 20, 23, 26, 35, 36, 38, 42, 43, 45, 55, 57, 59, 63, 64, 68, 69, 101, 104
DNA 12, 25, 30, 34, 35, 36, 37, 41, 45, 47, 51, 53
Ethics 10, 24, 100
Exome 34, 42
Exome sequencing 39, 43
Genome 23, 28, 34, 35, 42, 90
Genome Editing 23
Genome editing 13
Genome research 8, 13, 22, 25, 27, 28, 30, 35, 38, 39, 40, 41, 42, 43, 44, 45, 46, 50, 58
Genomics 18, 25, 26, 27, 29, 37, 39, 60, 91, 101, 102, 103

Gene therapies 27, 40, 43, 46, 90, 91, 97, 102
Health data 55, 59
Health policy 11
Guanine 35
Hepatitis 88, 89
Herpes viruses 88
Cardiovascular diseases 12, 15, 19, 26, 39, 49, 58, 59, 60, 67
HIV 15, 88, 89, 90, 103
High-throughput sequencing 25, 34, 38, 42, 47
High-throughput sequencing technologies 29
Human genome project 13, 28, 29, 30
Immunology 79, 90, 91
Immunotherapy 8, 13, 23, 77, 78, 79, 80, 81, 84, 85, 86, 87, 88, 90, 101, 103
Infectiology 40, 103
Infectious diseases 11, 15, 19
Intensive care 67
Ivacaftor 44, 49
Germline modifications 51, 102
KI 9, 13, 20, 22, 23, 55, 56, 57, 58, 59, 60, 61, 62, 63, 64, 65, 66, 67, 68, 69, 70, 71, 72, 73, 74, 75, 101, 103, 104
Climate change 16
Cancer 13, 15, 19, 20, 25, 26, 27, 32, 64, 69, 77, 79, 84
Cancer medicine 39
Cancer therapy 31, 47
Artificial intelligence 9, 18, 22
Luxturna 40, 44
Malaria 15
Mammography 64, 69
medical imaging 63, 64
Molecular biology 12, 79, 90
Monoclonal antibodies 77, 78, 82
Cystic fibrosis 44, 48
Mutation 27
Sustainability 10, 17
Neurodegenerative diseases 15
NGS 34, 35, 36, 37, 42, 47
Oncology 9, 27, 29, 36, 55, 58, 60, 63, 66, 81
Parkinson's 21
Personalised medicine 13, 15, 28, 35, 46, 47, 48, 49, 50, 59
Pharmacogenomics 27, 37, 40, 48, 60, 66

prenatal diagnoses 45
Prevention 9, 11, 16, 30, 38, 46, 59, 101
Proteomics 91, 102
Rehabilitation 67
Resistance 21
Screening 16, 39, 69
Sickle cell anaemia 31, 40, 44, 48, 51
Thymine 35
Transcriptome 34
Transplantation medicine 41
Trisomy 21 42, 45

Tuberculosis 15, 88, 89, 103
Tumour genomes 39
T cells 78, 79, 80, 81, 82, 83, 84, 85, 87, 93, 94, 97, 103
Environmental factors 29, 50
Responsibility 72, 73, 74, 97, 99
Virology 16
Accessibility 10, 23, 56, 57, 91, 95, 97, 105
Cytokines 80